PHYSICAL THERAPIST ASSISTANT

BY

ALFAJIRI PUBLISHERS

ALFAJIRI PUBLICATIONS
1510 WEST PAWNEE
WICHITA, KANSAS

TABLE OF CONTENTS

INTRODUCTION TO ANATOMY

Skeletal System

When many people imagine anatomy, they think of a skeleton. Your skeletal system is made up of your bones. Bones give your body the structure and shape it needs to move. They also help to protect your soft internal organs. Your bones have a hard, powerful outer surface made of compact material that can withstand forces, and they have a jelly-like interior called bone marrow. There are 206 bones within an adult's body. In order to grow, bones need calcium, which can be found in milk.

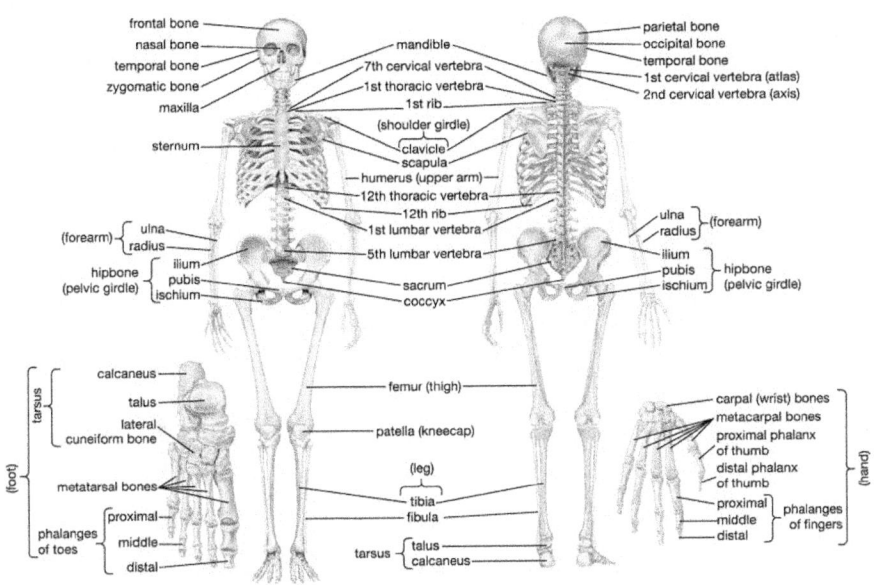

Muscular System

Muscles are made up of bundles of long, thin cells. Your body's motions come from muscles either contracting or relaxing. The muscles that move bones, such as in your arm, work in pairs together to produce movement. For example, as you raise your forearm, the muscle at the front of your upper arm, your bicep, contracts and forms a bulge. As you let your forearm back down, your tricep on the back of your upper arm will contract and your bicep will relax. In order to become stronger, people exercise. That exercise leads to tiny micro-tears in the fibers, which heal and become stronger.

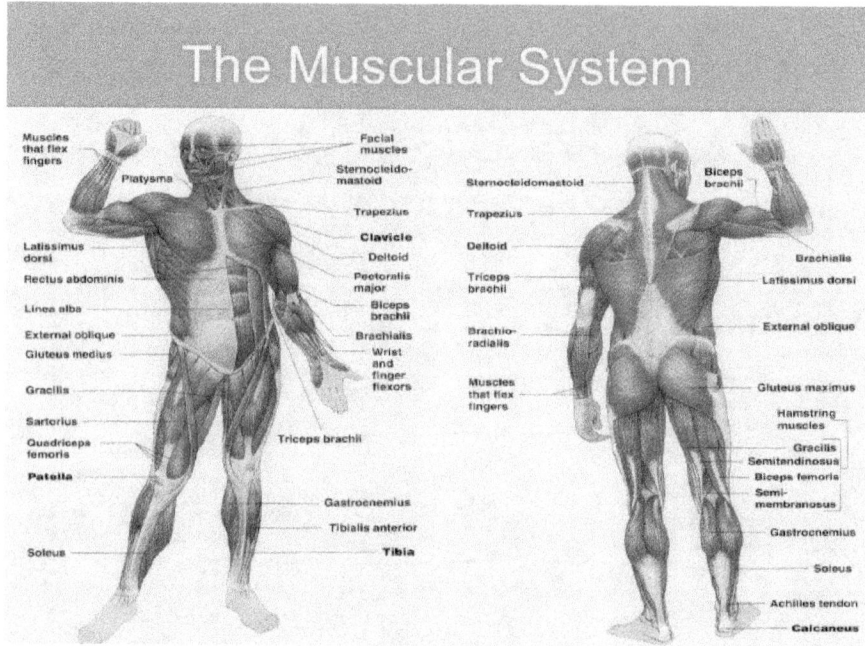

Cardiovascular System

Your heart is a muscle, but it's also part of its own system: the cardiovascular system. Your heart's job is to pump blood, which will circulate throughout the body. Blood is pumped through arteries and capillaries and comes back to the heart through veins. Your heart is always working, so it's important to take proper care of it by exercising and eating well.

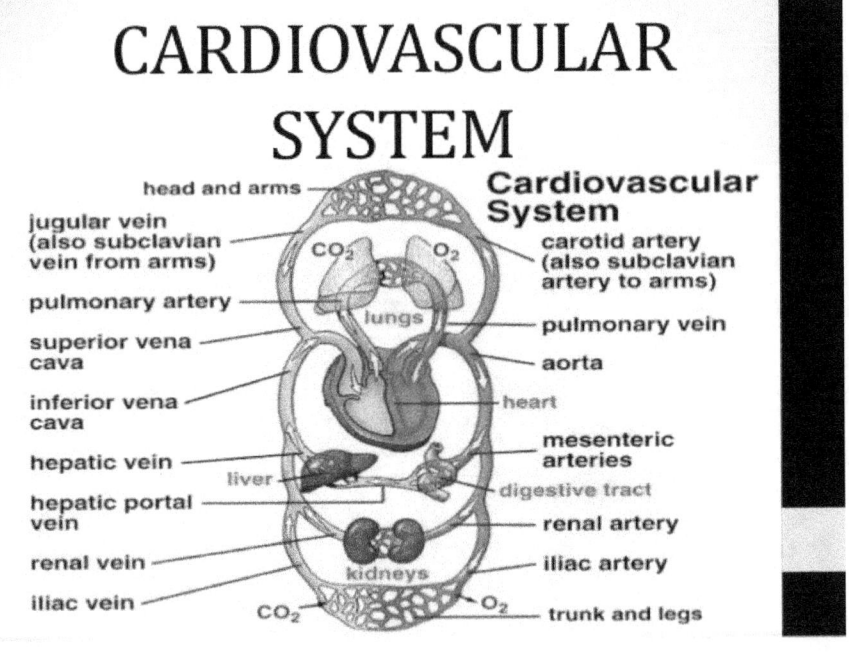

Digestive System

Your digestive system is very important and includes many different organs. Food travels from your mouth through your esophagus to your stomach, then into your intestines and your rectum. As it moves throughout the body, the food is digested. In other words, useable nutrients are absorbed into the bloodstream, and waste is disposed of as feces.

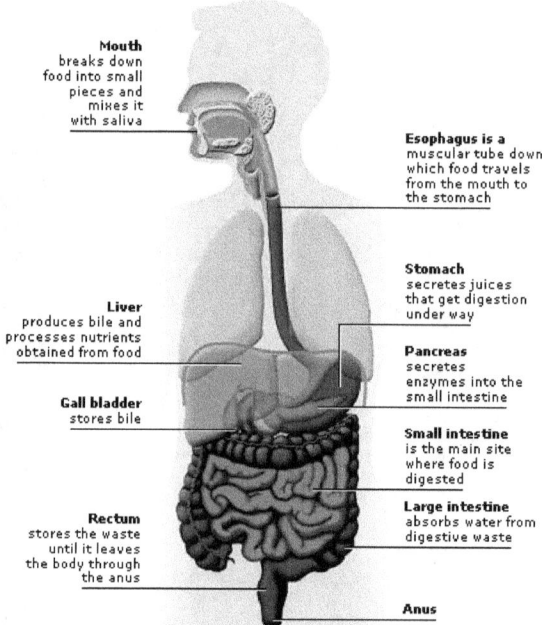

Mouth
breaks down food into small pieces and mixes it with saliva

Esophagus is a muscular tube down which food travels from the mouth to the stomach

Stomach secretes juices that get digestion under way

Liver produces bile and processes nutrients obtained from food

Pancreas secretes enzymes into the small intestine

Gall bladder stores bile

Small intestine is the main site where food is digested

Rectum stores the waste until it leaves the body through the anus

Large intestine absorbs water from digestive waste

Anus

Respiratory System

Your body needs oxygen to function. The organs that are responsible for taking in and processing the air are part of the respiratory system. Those organs include the pharynx, larynx, trachea, bronchial tubes, and lungs. The lungs have a hard job to do: They absorb oxygen so that it can be sent to the heart and circulated throughout the body. The lungs can be harmed when breathing in bad chemicals, such as from cigarettes.

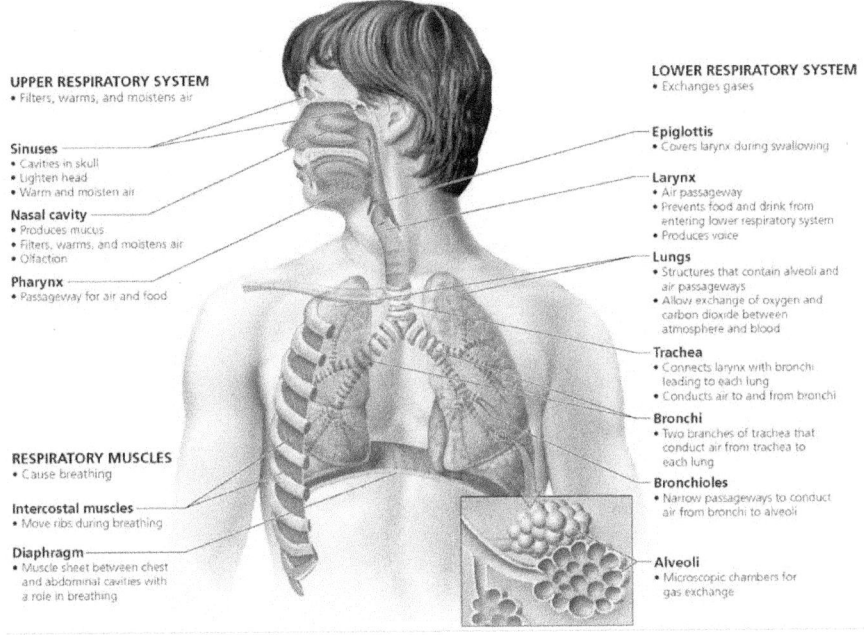

UPPER RESPIRATORY SYSTEM
• Filters, warms, and moistens air

Sinuses
• Cavities in skull
• Lighten head
• Warm and moisten air

Nasal cavity
• Produces mucus
• Filters, warms, and moistens air
• Olfaction

Pharynx
• Passageway for air and food

RESPIRATORY MUSCLES
• Cause breathing

Intercostal muscles
• Move ribs during breathing

Diaphragm
• Muscle sheet between chest and abdominal cavities with a role in breathing

LOWER RESPIRATORY SYSTEM
• Exchanges gases

Epiglottis
• Covers larynx during swallowing

Larynx
• Air passageway
• Prevents food and drink from entering lower respiratory system
• Produces voice

Lungs
• Structures that contain alveoli and air passageways
• Allow exchange of oxygen and carbon dioxide between atmosphere and blood

Trachea
• Connects larynx with bronchi leading to each lung
• Conducts air to and from bronchi

Bronchi
• Two branches of trachea that conduct air from trachea to each lung

Bronchioles
• Narrow passageways to conduct air from bronchi to alveoli

Alveoli
• Microscopic chambers for gas exchange

Nervous System

In addition to containing a vast network of arteries, veins, muscles, and bones, your body also contains a network of nerves, which touch almost every part of the body. The system can be broken up into two major systems: the central nervous system and the peripheral nervous system. The central nervous system contains the brain and spinal cord, which is the epicenter of nerve cells. Outside of that region is the peripheral nervous system where nerves often connect with other muscles and tissues. As human beings, we have fairly big brains, which allow us to read, think, and react to things.

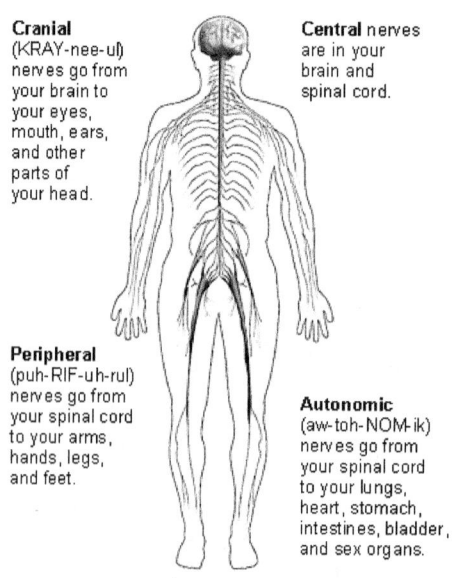

Cranial (KRAY-nee-ul) nerves go from your brain to your eyes, mouth, ears, and other parts of your head.

Central nerves are in your brain and spinal cord.

Peripheral (puh-RIF-uh-rul) nerves go from your spinal cord to your arms, hands, legs, and feet.

Autonomic (aw-toh-NOM-ik) nerves go from your spinal cord to your lungs, heart, stomach, intestines, bladder, and sex organs.

Excretory System

The excretory system is similar to the digestive system in that it's responsible for discharging wastes. The difference is that the excretory system gets rid of liquid waste. This system is responsible for keeping the chemical balance in the bloodstream. Related organs include the kidneys, skin, and bladder. Through urine and sweat, waste is excreted.

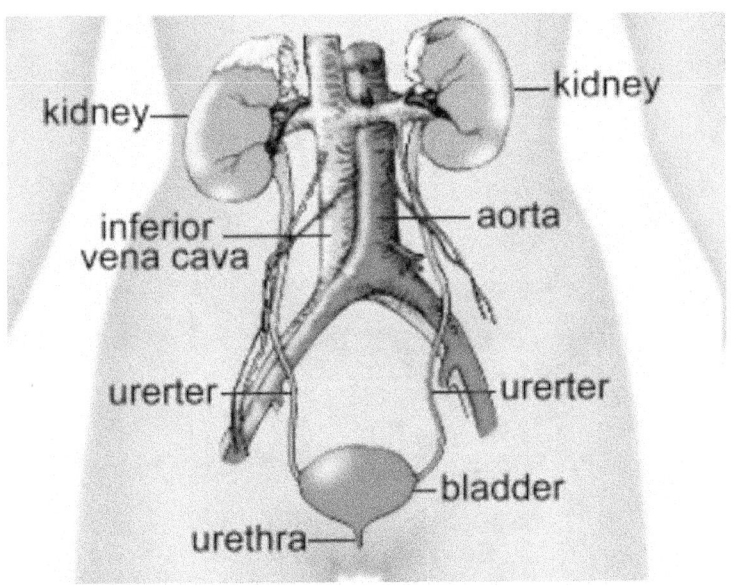

Humans Excretory System

Endocrine System

Growing up, you may hear a lot about hormones. Hormones are related to the endocrine system, which consists of a group of organs that communicate with chemical messages. There are quite a few organs in this system, all with their own unique chemical signature: the pineal gland, pituitary gland, hypothalamus, thymus, thyroid, adrenal glands, pancreas, and sex glands. This is one of the least-understood systems of the body, but we do know that these organs release chemicals into the bloodstream to let the rest of the body know what to do.

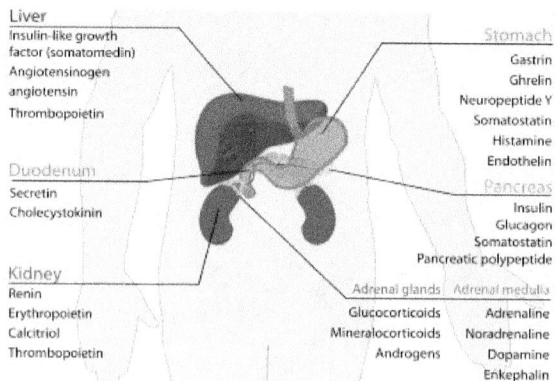

Liver
Insulin-like growth
factor (somatomedin)
Angiotensinogen
angiotensin
Thrombopoietin

Duodenum
Secretin
Cholecystokinin

Kidney
Renin
Erythropoietin
Calcitriol
Thrombopoietin

Stomach
Gastrin
Ghrelin
Neuropeptide Y
Somatostatin
Histamine
Endothelin

Pancreas
Insulin
Glucagon
Somatostatin
Pancreatic polypeptide

Adrenal glands
Glucocorticoids
Mineralocorticoids
Androgens

Adrenal medulla
Adrenaline
Noradrenaline
Dopamine
Enkephalin

ANATOMY QUIZ

1) Which of the following terms describes the body's ability to maintain its normal state?

(A) Anabolism
(B) Catabolism
(C) Tolerance
(D) Homeostasis
(E) Metabolism

2) Which of the following best describes the human body's defense mechanism against environmental bacteria?

(A) Hair in the nose
(B) Mucous membranes
(C) Osteoblasts
(D) Saliva
(E) Tears

3) Which of the following best describes a nucleus cell?

(A) Lymphocyte
(B) Monocyte
(C) Erythrocyte
(D) Basophil
(E) Neutrophil

4) Which of the following is flexible connective tissue that is attached to bones at the joints?

(A) Adipose
(B) Cartilage
(C) Epithelial
(D) Muscle
(E) Nerve

5) Which of the following allows air to pass into the lungs?

(A) Aorta
(B) Esophagus
(C) Heart

(D) Pancreas

(E) Trachea

6) Which of the following is the body cavity that contains the pituitary gland?

(A) Abdominal

(B) Cranial

(C) Pleural

(D) Spinal

(E) Thoracic

7) Which of the following closes and seals off the lower airway during swallowing?

(A) Alveoli

(B) Epiglottis

(C) Larynx

(D) Uvula

(E) Vocal cords

8) Which of the following is located beneath the diaphragm in the left upper quadrant of the abdominal cavity?

(A) Appendix

(B) Kidney

(C) Liver

(D) Spleen

(E) Stomach

9) Which of the following anatomical regions of abdomen lies just distal to the sternum?

(A) Epigastric

(B) Hypochondriac

(C) Hypogastric

(D) Lumbar

(E) Umbilical

10) Which of the following cavities are separated by the diaphragm?

(A) Abdominal and pelvic

(B) Cranial and spinal

(C) Dorsal and ventral

(D) Pericardial and pleural

(E) Thoracic and abdominal

11) Which of the following terms describes the motion of bending the forearm toward the body?

(A) Abduction
(B) Eversion
(C) Flexion
(D) Pronation
(E) Supination

12) In which of the following positions does a patient lie face down?

(A) Dorsal
(B) Erect
(C) Lateral
(D) Prone
(E) Supine

13) If the foot is abducted, it is moved in which direction?

(A) Inward
(B) Outward
(C) Upward
(D) Downward

14) The anatomic location of the spinal canal is

(A) caudal
(B) dorsal
(C) frontal
(D) transverse
(E) ventral

15) Which of the following is a structural, fibrous protein found in the dermis?

(A) Collagen
(B) Heparin
(C) Lipocyte
(D) Melanin
(E) Sebum

16) A patient has a fracture in which the radius is bent but not displaced, and the skin is intact. This type of fracture is known as which of the following?

(A) Closed, greenstick
(B) Complex, comminuted
(C) Compound, transverse
(D) Open, spiral
(E) Simple, pathologic

17) Which of the following is the large bone found superior to the patella and inferior to the ischium?

(A) Calcaneus
(B) Femur
(C) Symphysis pubis
(D) Tibia
(E) Ulna

18) The physician directs the medical assistant to complete a request form for an X-ray study of the fibula. The procedure will be performed on which of the following structures?

(A) Heel
(B) Lower leg
(C) Toes
(D) Thigh
(E) Pelvis

19) Which of the following is a disorder characterized by uncontrollable episodes of falling asleep during the day?

(A) Dyslexia
(B) Epilepsy
(C) Hydrocephalus
(D) Narcolepsy
(E) Shingles

20) Which of the following is the point at which an impulse is transmitted from one neuron to another neuron?

(A) Dendrite
(B) Glial cell
(C) Nerve center
(D) Synapse
(E) Terminal plate

21) Which of the following controls body temperature, sleep, and appetite?

(A) Adrenal glands
(B) Hypothalamus
(C) Pancreas
(D) Thalamus
(E) Thyroid gland

22) Which of the following cranial nerves is related to the sense of smell?

(A) Abducens
(B) Hypoglossal
(C) Olfactory
(D) Trochlear
(E) Vagus

23) Which of the following is a substance that aids the transmission of nerve impulses to the muscles?

(A) Acetylcholine
(B) Cholecystokinin
(C) Deoxyribose
(D) Oxytocin
(E) Prolactin

24) Which of the following best describes the location where the carotid pulse can be found?

(A) In front of the ears and just above eye level
(B) In the antecubital space
(C) In the middle of the groin
(D) On the anterior side of the neck
(E) On the medial aspect of the wrist

25) A patient sustains severe blunt trauma to the left upper abdomen and requires surgery. Which one of the following organs is most likely to be involved?

(A) Appendix
(B) Gallbladder
(C) Pancreas
(D) Urinary bladder
(E) Spleen

26) Where is the sinoatrial node located?

(A) Between the left atrium and the left ventricle
(B) Between the right atrium and the right ventricle
(C) In the interventricular septum
(D) In the upper wall of the left ventricle
(E) In the upper wall of the right atrium

27) Blood flows from the right ventricle of the heart into which of the following structures?

(A) Inferior vena cava
(B) Left ventricle
(C) Pulmonary arteries
(D) Pulmonary veins
(E) Right atrium

28) Oxygenated blood is carried to the heart by which of the following structures?

(A) Aorta
(B) Carotid arteries
(C) Inferior vena cava
(D) Pulmonary veins
(E) Superior vena cava

29) The thoracic cage is a structural unit important for which of the following functions?

(A) Alimentation
(B) Menstruation
(C) Mentation
(D) Respiration
(E) Urination

30) Which of the following substances is found in greater quantity in exhaled air?

(A) Carbon dioxide
(B) Carbon monoxide
(C) Nitrogen
(D) Oxygen
(E) Ozone

31) Which of the following allows gas exchange in the lungs?

(A) Alveoli
(B) Bronchi
(C) Bronchioles

(D) Capillaries

(E) Pleurae

32) At which of the following locations does bile enter the digestive tract?

(A) Gastroesophageal sphincter

(B) Duodenum

(C) Ileocecum

(D) Jejunum

(E) Pyloric sphincter

33) Which of the following structures is part of the small intestine?

(A) Ascending colon

(B) Cecum

(C) Ileum

(D) Sigmoid colon

(E) Transverse colon

34) Which of the following conditions is characterized by incompetence of the esophageal sphincter?

(A) Crohn's disease

(B) Esophageal varices

(C) Gastroesophageal reflux disease

(D) Pyloric stenosis

(E) Stomatitis

35) Which of the following organs removes bilirubin from the blood, manufactures plasma proteins, and is involved with the production of prothrombin and fibrinogen?

(A) Gallbladder

(B) Kidney

(C) Liver

(D) Spleen

(E) Stomach

36) Which of the following is an accessory organ of the gastrointestinal system that is responsible for secreting insulin?

(A) Adrenal gland

(B) Gallbladder

(C) Liver

(D) Pancreas

(E) Spleen

37) Which of the following is the lymphoid organ that is a reservoir for red blood cells and filters organisms from the blood?

(A) Appendix

(B) Gallbladder

(C) Pancreas

(D) Spleen

(E) Thymus

38) Which of the following best describes the process whereby the stomach muscles contract to propel food through the digestive tract?

(A) Absorption

(B) Emulsion

(C) Peristalsis

(D) Regurgitation

(E) Secretion

39) Saliva contains an enzyme that acts upon which of the following nutrients?

(A) Starches

(B) Proteins

(C) Fats

(D) Minerals

(E) Vitamins

40) In men, specimens for gonococcal cultures are most commonly obtained from which of the following structures?

(A) Anus

(B) Bladder

(C) Skin

(D) Testicle

(E) Urethra

41) Which of the following describes the cluster of blood capillaries found in each nephron in the kidney?

(A) Afferent arteriole

(B) Glomerulus

(C) Loop of Henle
(D) Renal pelvis
(E) Renal tubule

42) Which of the following conditions is characterized by the presence of kidney stones (renal calculi)?

(A) Glomerulonephritis
(B) Interstitial nephritis
(C) Nephrolithiasis
(D) Polycystic kidney
(E) Pyelonephritis

43) Which of the following best describes the structure that collects urine in the body?

(A) Bladder
(B) Kidney
(C) Ureter
(D) Urethra
(E) Urethral meatus

44) In men, which of the following structures is located at the neck of the bladder and surrounds the urethra?

(A) Epididymis
(B) Prostate
(C) Scrotum
(D) Seminal vesicle
(E) Vas deferens

45) Male hormones are produced by which of the following?

(A) Glans penis
(B) Prepuce
(C) Prostate
(D) Testes
(E) Vas deferens

46) Which of the following are mucus-producing glands located on each side of the vaginal opening?

(A) Adrenal
(B) Bartholin's

(C) Bulbourethral

(D) Corpus luteum

(E) Parotid

47) Fertilization of an ovum by a spermatozoon occurs in which of the following structures?

(A) Cervix

(B) Fallopian tube

(C) Ovary

(D) Uterus

(E) Vagina

48) Calcium, potassium, and sodium are classified as which of the following?

(A) Androgens

(B) Catecholamines

(C) Electrolytes

(D) Estrogens

(E) Prostaglandins

49) Which of the following is the master gland of the endocrine system?

(A) Adrenal

(B) Pancreas

(C) Pineal

(D) Pituitary

(E) Thyroid

50) Patients with which of the following diseases are treated with injections of vitamin B-12?

(A) Bell's palsy

(B) Crohn's disease

(C) Diabetes mellitus

(D) Graves' disease

(E) Pernicious anemia

ANATOMY ANSWERS

1) D

2) B

3) C

4) B

5) E

6) B

7) B

8) C

9) A

10) E

11) C

12) D

13) B

14) B

15) A

16) A

17) B

18) B

19) D

20) D

21) B

22) C

23) A

24) D

25) E

26) E

27) C

28) D

29) D

30) A

31) A

32) B

33) C

34) C

35) C

36) D

37) D

38) C

39) A

40) E

41) B

42) C

43) A

44) B

45) D

46) B

47) B

48) C

49) D

50) E

ABBREVIATIONS

A

@ – at

ā – before

A: – assessment

AAA – abdominal aortic aneurysm

AAROM – active assistive range of motion

Abd. or abd. – abduction

ABG – arterial blood gas

ABI – acquired brain injury

ac – before meals

AC – acromioclavicular

ACL – anterior cruciate ligament

ACTH – adrenocorticotropic hormone

Add. or add. – adduction

ADL's or ADL – activities of daily living

ad lib – at discretion

adm – admission/admitted

AE – above elbow

afib – atrial fibrillation

AFO – ankle foot orthosis

AIDS – acquired immune deficiency syndrome

AIIS – anterior inferior iliac spine

AJ – ankle jerk

AK – above knee

AKA – above knee amputee, above knee amputation

ALS – amyotrophic lateral sclerosis

a.m. – morning

AMA – against medical advice

amb – ambulate, ambulates, ambulated, ambulatory, ambulation

ANS – autonomic nervous system

Ant. – anterior

AP – anterior-posterior

approx. – approximately (also "~" symbol can be used)

ARDS – adult respiratory distress syndrome

ARF – acute renal failure

AROM – active range of motion

AROME - active range of motion exercise/s

ASA – aspirin

ASAP or asap – as soon as possible

ASCVD – arteriosclerotic cardiovascular disease

ASHD – arteriosclerotic heart disease

ASIS – anterior superior iliac spine

Assist. – assistive, assistance

A-V – arteriovenous

AVM – arteriovenous malformation

B

B/S – bedside

BE – below elbow

bed mob. – bed mobility

BID or bid – twice a day

bilat – bilateral (a B enclosed within a circle may also be used)

BK – below knee

BKA – below knee amputee, below knee amputation

BM – bowel movement

BOS – base of support

BP – blood pressure

bpm – beats per minute

BR – bedrest

BRP – bathroom privileges

BS – breath sounds/bowel sounds

BLE – both lower extremities

BUE – both upper extremities

BUN – blood urea nitrogen

C

c̄ - with

C&S – culture and sensitivity

c/o – complains of

CA – cancer, carcinoma

CABG – coronary artery bypass graft

CAD – coronary artery disease

CAT – computerized axial tomography

CBC – complete blood count

C/C – chief complaint

cc. – cubic centimeter

cerv. - cervical

CF – cystic fibrosis

CHF – congestive heart failure

CHI – closed head injury

CKD – chronic kidney disease

cm. – centimeter

CMV – cytomegalovirus

CNS – central nervous system

CO – cardiac output

CO2 – carbon dioxide

Cont. or cont. – continue

COPD – chronic obstructive pulmonary disease

COTA – certified occupational therapist assistant

CP – cerebral palsy

CPAP – continuous positive airway pressure

CPR – cardiopulmonary resuscitation

CRF – chronic renal failure

CSF – cerebrospinal fluid

CV – cardiovascular

CVD – cardiovascular disease

CWI – crutch walking instructions

CXR – chest x-ray

Cysto – cystoscopic examination

D

D/C – discontinue, discontinued, discharge, discharged

dept. – department

DF - dorsiflexion

DIP – distal interphalangeal

DJD – degenerative joint disease

DM – diabetes mellitus

DNR – do not resuscitate

DO – doctor of osteopathy

DOB – date of birth

DOE – dyspnea on exertion

DTR – deep tendon reflex

DVT – deep vein thrombosis

Dx – diagnosis

E

ECF – extended care facility (In Physiology – extracellular fluid)

ECG/EKG – electrocardiogram, electrocardiograph

ED – emergency department

EEG – electroencephalogram, electroencephalograph

EENT – ear, eyes, nose, throat

EMG – electromyogram, electromyography, electromyography

ER or Ext. rot. – external rotation

E.R. – emergency room

eval. – evaluation

Ex. – exercise

ext. – extension

F

FBS – fasting blood sugar

FEV – forced expiratory volume

FH – family history

flex. – flexion

FRC – functional residual capacity

FUO – fever unknown origin

FVC – forced vital capacity

FWB – full weight bearing

Fx., fx – fracture

G

GB – gall bladder

GCS – Glasgow coma scale

GI – gastrointestinal

GIT – gastrointestinal tract

GSW – gunshot wound

GYN – gynecology

H

H/A - headache

H&H, H/H – hematocrit and hemoglobin

Hct – hematocrit

HEENT – head, ear, eyes, nose, throat

Hemi. – hemiplegia, hemiparesis

HEP – home exercise program

Hgb – hemoglobin

HIV – human immunodeficiency virus

HKAFO – hip knee ankle foot orthosis

HNP – herniated nucleus pulposus

h/o – history of

HOB – head of bed

HR – heart rate

hr. - hour

hs – at bedtime

HTN or Htn – hypertension

Hx – history

I

I&O – intake and output

IADL – instrumental activities of daily living

ICU – intensive care unit

IDDM – insulin dependent diabetes mellitus

IE – <u>initial evaluation</u>

IFC – interferential current

IM – intramuscular

imp. – impression

indep – independent

inf. – inferior

inv. - inversion

IR or int. rot. – internal rotation

IRDS – infant respiratory distress syndrome

IS – incentive spirometer, incentive spirometry

IV – intravenous

K

KAFO – knee ankle foot orthosis

kcal – kilocalories

KJ – knee jerk

KUB – kidney, ureter, bladder

L

L within a circle – left

Lat – lateral

LBBB – left bundle branch block

LBP – <u>low back pain</u>

LE – lower extremity

LOC – loss of consciousness, level of consciousness

LMN – lower motor neuron

LMNL – lower motor neuron lesion

LOS – length of stay

LP – lumbar puncture

LLQ – left lower quadrant

LQ – lower quadrant

LTG – long term goal

LUQ – left upper quadrant

M

MAP – mean arterial pressure

max. – maximal

MD – medical doctor, doctor of medicine

MED – minimal erythemal dose

Meds. – medications

MI – myocardial infarction

min – minimal

min. – minute

mm. - muscle

MMT – manual muscle test, manual muscle testing

mod. – moderate

MP – metacarpophalangeal

MRSA – methicilin resistant staphylococcus virus

MS – multiple sclerosis

MVA – motor vehicle accident

N

NDT – neurodevelopmental treatment

neg. – negative

NG or ng – nasogastric

N.H. – nursing home

NIDDM – non-insulin dependent diabetes mellitus

nn. – nerve

noc – night, at night

NPO or npo – nothing by mouth

NSR – normal sinus rhythm

NWB – non-weight bearing

O

O: - objective

OA – osteoarthritis

OB – obstetrics

OBS – organic brain syndrome

od – once daily

OOB – out of bed

O.P. – outpatient

O.R. – operating room

ORIF – open reduction, internal fixation

OT – occupational therapist/therapy

OTR – registered occupational therapist

P

$\overline{p}$ – after

P – poor (used in muscle testing)

P: - plan

P.A. – physician's assistant

PA – posterior/anterior

para – paraplegia

pc – after meals

PCL – posterior cruciate ligament

PE – pulmonary embolus

PEEP – positive end expiratory pressure

per – by/through

PF – plantar flexion

p.o. – by mouth (per orem)

PERRLA – pupils equal, round, reactive to light and accommodation

P.H. – past history

p.m. – afternoon

PMH – past medical history

PNF – proprioceptive neuromuscular facilitation

PNI – peripheral nerve injury

POMR – problem-oriented medical record

pos. - positive

poss – possible

post. – posterior

post-op – after surgery

PRE – progressive resistive exercise

pre-op – before operation

Prep. – preparation

prn – whenever necessary

PROM – passive range of motion

PROME – passive range of motion exercise

PSIS – posterior superior iliac spine

PT – physical therapy/ therapist

PT – prothrombin time

Pt. or pt. – patient

PTA – prior to admission

PTA – physical therapist assistant

PTB – patellar tendon bearing

PVD – peripheral vascular disease

PWB – partial weight bearing

Q

q – every

qd – everyday

qh – ever hour

qid – four times a day

qn – every night

R

® - right

RA – rheumatoid arthritis

RBBB – right bundle branch block

R.D. – registered dietitian

Rehab – rehabilitation

reps. – repetitions

resp – respiratory, respiration

RN – registered nurse

R/O or r/o – rule out

ROM – range of motion

ROME – range of motion exercises

ROS – review of systems

rot. – rotation

RR – respiratory rate

RROM – resistive range of motion

R.T. – respiratory therapist/therapy

Rx – prescription; therapy; intervention plan; treatment

S

$\overline{s}$ – without

SACH – solid ankle cushion heel

SBA – standby assist

SCI – spinal cord injury

SC jt. – sternoclavicular joint

SED – suberythemal dose

sig – directions for use; use as follows; let it be labeled

SI jt. – sacroiliac joint

SLE – systemic lupus erythematosus

SLP – speech-language pathologist

SLR – straight leg raise

SNF – skilled nursing facility

SOAP – subjective, objective, assessment, plan

SOB – shortness of breath

S/P – status post

S/Sx – signs and symptoms

stat. – immediately or at once

STG – short term goal

sup. – superior

Sx – symptoms

T

tab – tablet

TB – tuberculosis

TBI – traumatic brain injury

TENS or TNS – transcutaneous electrical nerve stimulator/ stimulation

THA – total hip arthroplasty

THR – total hip replacement

TIA – transient ischemic attack

tid – three times daily

TIW – three times per week

TKA – total knee arthroplasty

TKR – total knee replacement

TMJ – temporomandibular joint

TNR – tonic neck reflex

t.o. – telephone order

TPR – temperature, pulse and respiration

TTWB – toe touch weight bearing

TV – tidal volume

Tx – treatment

tx – traction

U

UA – urine analysis

UE – upper extremity

UMN – upper motor neuron

UMNL – upper motor neuron lesion

URI – upper respiratory infection

US - ultrasound

UTI – urinary tract infection

UV ultraviolet

V

VC – vital capacity

VC – verbal cues

VD – venereal disease

VO or v.o. – verbal orders

Vol. – volume

v.s. – vital signs

W

w/c – wheel chair

W/cm2 – watts per centimeter square

WBC – white blood cell

WFL – within functional limits

wk. – week

WNL – within normal limits

wt. – weight

X

x – number of times performed (e.g. x3, x8, etc.)

Y

y/o or y.o. – years old

yr. – year

PT SYMBOLS

+1, +2 - assistance

♂ - male

♀ - female

↓ - down, downward, decrease, diminished

↑ - up, upward, increase

// - parallel, parallel bars (also // bars)

$\bar{c}$ - with

$\bar{s}$ - without

$\bar{p}$ - after

$\bar{a}$ - before

~ - approximately

@ - at

Δ - change

> - greater than

< - less than

= - equal

+ - positive

- - negative

- number (e.g., #1) or pounds (e.g., 5# wt.)

/ - per

% - percent

↔ - to and from

→ - to, progressing toward, approaching

1° - primary

2° - secondary, secondary to

CENTRAL NERVOUS SYSTEM

The Vertebrate Nervous System:

1 - receives stimuli from receptors & transmits information to effectors that respond to stimulation

2 - regulates behavior by integrating incoming sensory information with stored information (the results of past experience) & translating that into action by way of effectors

3 - includes billions of nerve cells (or neurons), each of which establishes thousands of contacts with other nerve cells

4 - also includes neuroglia cells that support, nourish, & insulate neurons

Subdivisions of the Vertebrate Nervous System:

1 - Central Nervous System - including the brain & spinal cord

2 - Peripheral Nervous System - including cranial nerves, spinal nerves, & all branches of cranial & spinal nerves

Neurons (or nerve cells):

- respond to stimuli & conduct impulses
- 3 types - all with cell body & processes (axons & dendrites):
  - multipolar
  - bipolar
  - unipolar

Spinal cord:

- located in vertebral canal
- anatomical beginning is the foramen magnum of the skull
- length varies among vertebrates:
  - in vertebrates with abundant tail musculature, the spinal cord extends to the caudal end of the vertebral column
  - in vertebrates without tails or without much tail musculature, the spinal cord extends to about the lumbar region of the vertebral column
- a cross-section of the spinal cord reveals gray matter & white matter. The gray matter consists of nerve cell bodies, while the white matter consists of nerve cell processes (axons). These processes make up ascending (sensory) and descending (motor) fiber tracts.

Spinal nerves:

- arise from spinal cord by dorsal & ventral roots. The dorsal root exhibits a ganglion & is sensory, while the ventral root has no ganglion & is motor.
- early vertebrates:
  - dorsal & ventral roots did not unite
  - dorsal roots were mixed (contained both sensory & motor fibers)
  - no dorsal root ganglion
- Rami - 2 branches of each spinal nerve:
  - dorsal ramus - supplies epaxial muscles & skin of the dorsal part of the body
  - ventral ramus - supplies hypaxial muscles & skin of the side & ventral part of the body
- Functional types of neurons in spinal nerves (& other nerves):
  - somatic afferent - sensory from general cutaneous receptors (in the skin) & proprioceptors (in skeletal muscles, tendons, & joints)
  - somatic efferent - motor to skeletal muscles
  - visceral afferent - sensory from receptors in the viscera (smooth muscle, cardiac muscle, & glands)
  - visceral efferent - motor to smooth muscle, cardiac muscle, & glands

Brain:

- the anterior end of the embryonic central nervous system exhibits 3 sections:
  - prosencephalon (forebrain) - subsequently divides into the telencephalon (cerebrum) & diencephalon (epithalamus, thalamus, & hypothalamus)
  - mesencephalon (midbrain) - develops without further subdivision & forms the tectum
  - rhombencephalon (hindbrain) - subdivides into the metencephalon (pons & cerebellum) and myelencephalon (medulla oblonga
- Phylogenetic trend in vertebrate brains is for enlargement of forebrain:
  - increasingly complex behaviors & muscle control:
    - coordination of limb movements more complicated (e.g., bipedal dinosaurs & birds)
    - increased input of sensory information & increased output of motor responses

Myelencephalon - consists of the medulla oblongata & its major functions include:

- origin of cranial nerves (VII - X or VII - XII)
- pathway for ascending & descending fiber tracts
- contains centers important in regulating respiration, heartbeat, & intestinal motility

Metencephalon - consists of the pons & cerebellum:

- Pons - pathway for ascending & descending fiber tracts & origin of cranial nerves V, VI, & VII
- Cerebellum - modifies & monitors motor output:
    - important in maintaining equilibrium
    - coordinates & refines motor action

Mesencephalon - consists of the tectum which includes the optic lobes & auditory lobes:

- optic lobes - receive fibers from retina; vary in size with relative importance of vision
- auditory lobes - receive fibers from inner ear

Diencephalon - consists of the epithalamus, hypothalamus, & thalamus:

- epithalamus - includes pineal gland (epiphysis) that affects skin pigmentation (by acting on melanocytes) in lower vertebrates & plays a role in regulating biological rhythms in higher vertebrates
- hypothalamus - regulates body temperature, water balance, appetite, blood pressure, sexual behavior, & some aspects of emotional behavior
- thalamus - major coordinating, or relay, center for sensory impulses from all parts of the body

ELECTRICAL STIMULATION

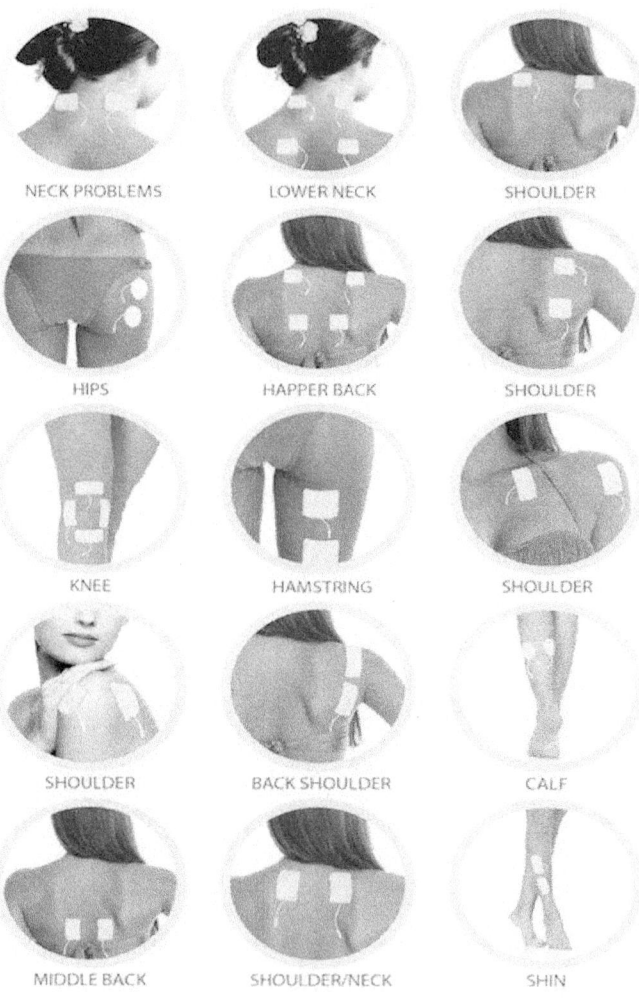

NECK PROBLEMS

LOWER NECK

SHOULDER

HIPS

HAPPER BACK

SHOULDER

KNEE

HAMSTRING

SHOULDER

SHOULDER

BACK SHOULDER

CALF

MIDDLE BACK

SHOULDER/NECK

SHIN

Electric stimulation therapy is a therapeutic treatment that applies electrical stimulation in treating muscle spasms and pain. It can help prevent atrophy and build strength in patients with injuries. It is also helpful in keeping muscles active especially after any type spinal cord injury or strokes.

Physical therapists and other medical practitioners attach electrodes on the patient's skin, causing the target muscles to contract. With electric stimulation, the patient can maintain muscle tone and strength that would otherwise waste away due to lack of usage.

Electric stimulation works by mimicking the natural way by which the body exercises its muscles. The electrodes attached to the skin deliver impulses that make the muscles contract. It is beneficial in increasing the patient's range of motion and improves the circulation of the body. It is used in treating conditions like sprains, arthritis, back pain scoliosis and sciatica.

Electric stimulation can be muscular, general and transcutaneous electrical nerve stimulation (TENS). The muscular type of electric stimulation seeks to strengthen the muscles by reducing muscle spasms. Also known as EMS, this stimulates the skeletal muscle using electric impulses to cause muscle contraction.

TENS is commonly used to help with chronic pain. The general type of electric stimulation is used for healing wounds and alleviating pain. For the convenience of the patient, a portable TENS unit can be prescribed by the doctor or a physical therapist for the patient to use at home.

Interferential current (IFC) is another form of TENS. It is used by physical therapists and chiropractors for the purpose of decreasing inflammation and swelling of affected tissues. This treatment has also shown positive effects in improving symptoms of asthma and in reducing back pain.

Galvanic stimulation is also another application of electric stimulation. This involves applying pulsed electric current on affected body tissues in stimulating muscle contraction. It differs with TENS and IFC in its use of direct current rather than alternating current. The positive pad acts to decrease circulation of the target area and reduce swelling. The negative pad increases the distribution of oxygen, blood and nutrients to the injured area thus increasing the speed of the healing process.

Administration of electric stimulation should exclude patients with pacemakers or those who have certain kinds of skin disease

Pregnant women should also avoid this treatment. As always, consulting certified medical practitioner should be done before using this treatment plan.

In using electric stimulation, physical therapists seek to improve quality of life for patients when the traditional treatment plans are not working.

Preamble

Physical Therapist Assistants are responsible for maintaining and promoting high standards of conduct. These Standards of Ethical Conduct for the Physical Therapist Assistant shall be binding on Physical Therapist Assistants who are affiliate members of the Association.

Standard 1
Physical Therapist Assistants provide services under the supervision of a Physical Therapist.

Standard 2
Physical Therapist Assistants respect the rights and dignity of all individuals.

Standard 3
Physical Therapist Assistants maintain and promote high standards in the provision of services giving the welfare of the patients their highest regard.

Standard 4
Physical Therapist Assistants provide services within the limits of the law.

Standard 5
Physical Therapist Assistants make those judgments that are commensurate with their qualifications as Physical Therapist Assistants.

Standard 6
Physical Therapist Assistants accept the responsibility to protect the public and the profession from unethical, incompetent, or illegal acts.

EXERCISES

Physical Therapy nearly always involves exercise of some kind that is specifically designed for your injury, illness, condition, or to help prevent future health problems.
Exercise is anything you do in addition to your regular daily activity that will improve your flexibility, strength, coordination, or endurance. It even includes changing how you do your regular exercises to give you some health benefits. For example, if you park a little farther away from the door of the grocery store, the extra distance you walk is exercise. Also, exercise can include stretching to reduce stress on joints, core stability exercises to strengthen the muscles of your trunk (your back and abdomen) and hips, lifting weights to strengthen muscles, walking, doing water aerobics, and many other forms of activity. Your physical therapist is likely to teach you how to do an exercise program on your own at home so you can continue to work toward your fitness goals and prevent future problems.

Manual therapy

Manual therapy (sometimes called bodywork) is a general term for treatment performed mostly with the hands. The goals of manual therapy include relaxation, decreased pain, and increased flexibility.

Manual therapy can include:

- Massage- Pressure is applied to the soft tissues of the body, such as the muscles. Massage can help relax muscles, increase circulation, and ease pain in the soft tissues.
- Mobilization. Slow, measured movements are used to twist, pull, or push bones and joints into position. This can help loosen tight tissues around a joint and help with flexibility and alignment.
- Manipulation- Pressure is applied to a joint. It can be done with the hands or a special device. The careful, controlled force used on the joint can range from gentle to strong and from slow to rapid.

Education

Physical therapy almost always includes education and training in areas such as:

- Performing your daily tasks safely.
- Protecting your joints and avoiding reinjury.
- Using assistive devices such as crutches or wheelchairs.
- Doing home exercises designed to help with your injury or condition.
- Making your home safe for you if you have strength, balance, or vision problems.
- **Specialized treatments**
- In some locations, physical therapists are specially trained to be involved in other types of treatment, including:

- Vestibular rehabilitation, which helps your inner ear respond to changes in your body position. This is helpful if you have problems with vertigo, or a feeling that you or your surroundings are spinning or tilting when there is actually no movement. Rehabilitation (rehab) can help you get used to the problem so you know when to expect it. And rehab can train your body to know how to react.
- Wound care- Wounds that are very severe or don't heal well, often because of poor blood flow to the area, can require extensive care. This may include special cleaning and bandaging on a regular and long-term basis. Sometimes oxygen treatment or electrical stimulation is part of the treatment.
- Pelvic health- Physical therapists can provide instruction in exercises to help control incontinence or to relieve pelvic pain.
- Oncology (cancer care), to help if cancer or treatment for cancer uses you to have problems with movement.
- Decongestive lymphatic drainage, which is a special form of massage to help reduce swelling when the lymphatic system is not properly draining fluids from your tissues.

Other treatments

Other treatments include:

- Cold and ice, to relieve pain, swelling, and inflammation from injuries and other conditions such as arthritis. Ice can be used for up to 20 minutes at a time. In some cases, ice may be used several times a day. Some therapists also use cooling lotions or sprays.
- Heat, to help relax and heal your muscles and soft tissues by increasing blood circulation. This can be especially helpful if a joint is stiff from osteoarthritis or from being immobilized. Heat can also relax the muscles before exercise. But heat can also increase swelling in an injured area if it is used too soon.
- Ultrasound therapy, which uses high-pitched sound waves to ease muscle spasms and relax and warm muscles before exercise, to help relieve pain and inflammation, and to promote healing.

- Electrical stimulation. In general, this is the use of electrical current to create an effect in the body. Electrical stimulation is sometimes used at low levels to reduce the feeling of pain. It can also be used to cause muscles to contract (tense). And it is being studied as a way to help with healing of wounds and broken bones.
- Hydrotherapy (water therapy), which is a term from the past that means the use of water to treat a disease or to maintain health. The most common hydrotherapy now is water exercise.

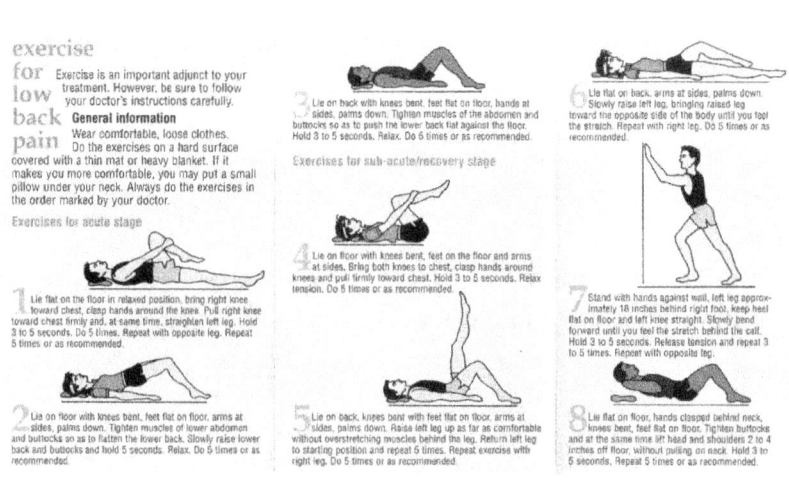

exercise for low back pain

Exercise is an important adjunct to your treatment. However, be sure to follow your doctor's instructions carefully.

General information

Wear comfortable, loose clothes. Do the exercises on a hard surface covered with a thin mat or heavy blanket. If it makes you more comfortable, you may put a small pillow under your neck. Always do the exercises in the order marked by your doctor.

Exercises for acute stage

1. Lie flat on the floor in relaxed position, bring right knee toward chest, clasp hands around the knee. Pull right knee toward chest firmly and, at same time, straighten left leg. Hold 3 to 5 seconds. Relax. Repeat with opposite leg. Repeat 5 times or as recommended.

2. Lie on floor with knees bent, feet flat on floor, arms at sides, palms down. Tighten muscles of lower abdomen and buttocks so as to flatten the lower back. Slowly raise lower back and buttocks and hold 5 seconds. Relax. Do 5 times or as recommended.

3. Lie on back with knees bent, feet flat on floor, hands at sides, palms down. Tighten muscles of the abdomen and buttocks so as to push the lower back flat against the floor. Hold 3 to 5 seconds. Relax. Do 5 times or as recommended.

Exercises for sub-acute/recovery stage

4. Lie on floor with knees bent, feet on the floor and arms at sides. Bring both knees to chest, clasp hands around knees and pull firmly toward chest. Hold 3 to 5 seconds. Relax tension. Do 5 times or as recommended.

5. Lie on back, knees bent with feet flat on floor, arms at sides, palms down. Raise left leg up as far as comfortable without overstretching muscles behind the leg. Return left leg to starting position and repeat 5 times. Repeat exercise with right leg. Do 5 times or as recommended.

6. Lie flat on back, arms at sides, palms down. Slowly raise left leg, bringing raised leg toward the opposite side of the body until you feel the stretch. Repeat with right leg. Do 5 times or as recommended.

7. Stand with hands against wall, left leg approximately 18 inches behind right foot, keep heel flat on floor and left knee straight. Slowly bend forward until you feel the stretch behind the calf. Hold 3 to 5 seconds. Release tension and repeat 3 to 5 times. Repeat with opposite leg.

8. Lie flat on floor, hands clasped behind neck, knees bent, feet flat on floor. Tighten buttocks and at the same time lift head and shoulders 2 to 4 inches off floor, without pulling on neck. Hold 3 to 5 seconds. Repeat 5 times or as recommended.

KNEE STRENGTH

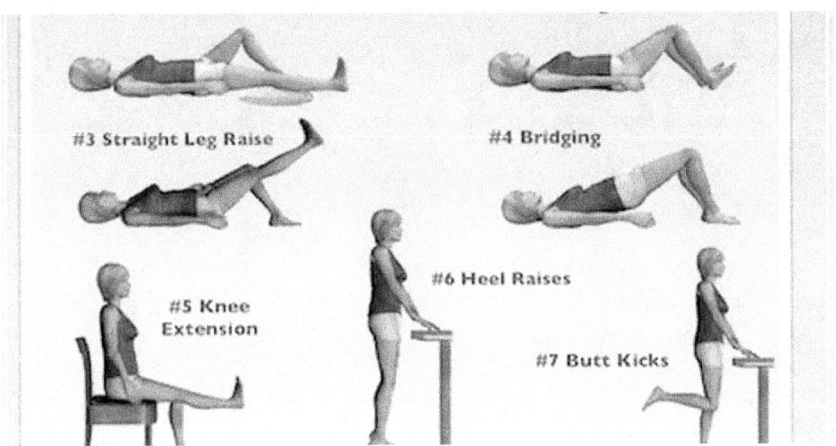

#3 Straight Leg Raise

#4 Bridging

#5 Knee Extension

#6 Heel Raises

#7 Butt Kicks

Neck Exercises

Neck Strain Exercises

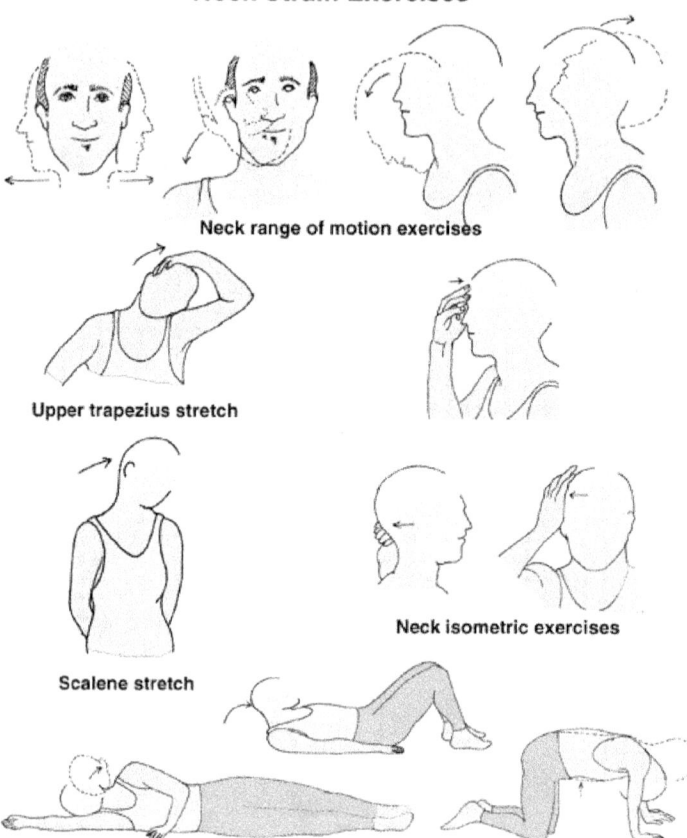

Neck range of motion exercises

Upper trapezius stretch

Neck isometric exercises

Scalene stretch

Head lifts

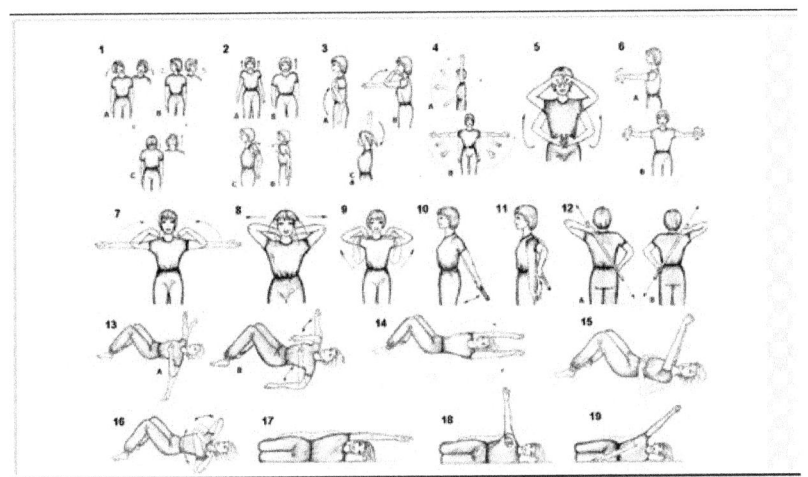

FLUID THERAPY
Treatment for Edema and Effusion

Simply put, swelling refers to an enlarged body part. Injuries often result in pain and swelling. At the same time, swelling can actually cause other injuries. Proper care after an injury can help reduce swelling and prevent further injuries. Physical Therapist can offer specific guidance for treating your injury and swelling.

Cause and Types of Swelling

The body part swells due to a chemical reaction within the body. When an injury occurs, there is a release of chemical agents that produce a response within the cells, making the cell wall more permeable. When the cell wall becomes more permeable and the pressure within the cell is greater than the pressure in the space between the cells (the interstitial space), the flow of fluid is along the gradient of higher to lower pressure. Therefore, the volume of fluid in the interstitial space increases along with the pressure. Eventually, the pressure in the interstitial space exceeds the pressure in the cells and the flow of fluid out of the cell is stopped.

There are two types of swelling: edema – swelling that occurs primarily in the soft tissues of the body and effusion – swelling or fluid in the joint space. Edema and effusion are a result of the change in the fluid levels in and out of the cells. Both edema and effusion compromise the body part, causing pain while reducing motion and strength.

Treatment of Edema or Effusion

The first line of treatment for such conditions is the RICE principles of acute injury care.

Rest

The first response to an injury and swelling should be rest. This removes strain off of affected area and prevents further injury. In some instances like a fracture, the involved area must be immobilized or significantly restricted with the use of splints, casts and braces.

Ice

By cooling the injured area, you can reduce the inflammatory response and pain. One by-product of the chemical reaction of inflammation is heat. Ice on the injury site extracts the fuel of heat and halt the inflammation.

Compression

The use of an ace-bandage to wrap the injury site and increase the pressure "outside" the cell helps to artificially increase the pressure within the interstitial space and help it surpass the pressure within the cell. Once the pressure is greater in the interstitial space, the fluid will stop moving across the high to low gradient from the cell to the space.

Elevation

If a body part accumulates an excess in fluid, gravity can force it to flow to an unrelated area of the body (i.e. the ankle when the knee is injured). If the injury site is elevated the excess in fluid will tend to "flow" towards the internal organs that are responsible for cleansing the blood and re-using anything that is re-usable and excreting the waste. The fluid returns to these organs via the lymphatic system.

Physical Therapy can also play a key role in treating edema and effusion. First, the Physical Therapist seeks to uncover the root cause of the edema or effusion. This diagnosis helps the therapist focus the exercise routine in a way that will help decrease the excess fluid in the area. Two great ways to reduce excess fluid in a body part is via muscle contraction and movement. Unless the diagnosis requires immobility, controlled motion can "force" or "pump" the fluid out of the injured area. The muscles in the injured area contract to move the joints and the fluid is moved towards the internal organs. The vessels have "one way" valves that open towards the organs and the muscle contraction "pumps" the fluid in that direction.

Seeking treatment from a Physical Therapist is easy and does not require the patient to see their doctor first. The Physical Therapist is a licensed professional who can evaluate and treat a patient without a doctor's prescription.

Effusion and Edema are similar in many ways and are usually "lumped" together in layman's terms as swelling. Regardless of the term used to describe the swelling the excess fluid that occurs needs to be addressed to restore normal function of the involved area.

FUNCTIONAL REHABILITATION

Condition: Functional rehabilitation combines various techniques in an attempt to return an injured athlete or worker to an optimal level of performance.

Background: The functional rehabilitation program includes strength, flexibility, and agility training as well as training focused on coordination of body parts and motion to prepare the individual to return to full participation.

Risk Factors: Typically, functional rehabilitation has been applied to sports medicine, but this approach is also beneficial for individuals returning to work or basic activities of daily living after traumatic injuries or even neurological injuries strokes.

History and Symptoms: History of the injury, including previous injuries, treatments, and recovery, is useful as the initial step. Understanding the patient's goals and plans to return to sports or activities is helpful. Knowledge of current level of function, presence of a support system, use of medications or supplements, and what positions or movements reduce or increase pain is also important.

Physical Exam: A physical examination will be performed to assess reflexes, posture, balance, walking, muscle control, body stabilization during rest and movement, range of motion of joints, and any deficiencies or problems that may have contributed to the original injury.

Diagnostic Process: Functional rehabilitation requires functional diagnostics, such as reviewing the athlete's techniques, movement capabilities, and secondary adaptation changes to other joints or muscles; however, imaging, such as X-ray, CT, or MRI, may be used to clarify the particular problem or injury. Ultrasound imaging can also be used to assess the movement of joints and muscles.

Rehab Management: The overall goal of functional rehabilitation is to train the patient using three-dimensional movements to prepare the whole body to return to daily activities or sports. This differs from therapies used to address the patient's symptoms using such modalities as heat, ice, and medication while mainly strengthening the isolated injured muscle. The athlete should begin rehabilitation as soon as the injury allows, and rehabilitation, which should be injury-specific, may follow a multi-phase program that involves progressive steps from controlling inflammation and pain to restoration of motion to development of muscle strength, power, and endurance to return to sport-specific activity. A team approach should involve rehabilitation physicians, physical therapists, athletic trainers, and strength and conditioning coaches.

Other Resources for Patients and Families: Patient's families and coaches should be educated about the training required for restoration of full function and for avoiding re-injury, as treatment failure often stems from returning to competition before full recovery.

GAIT TRAINING

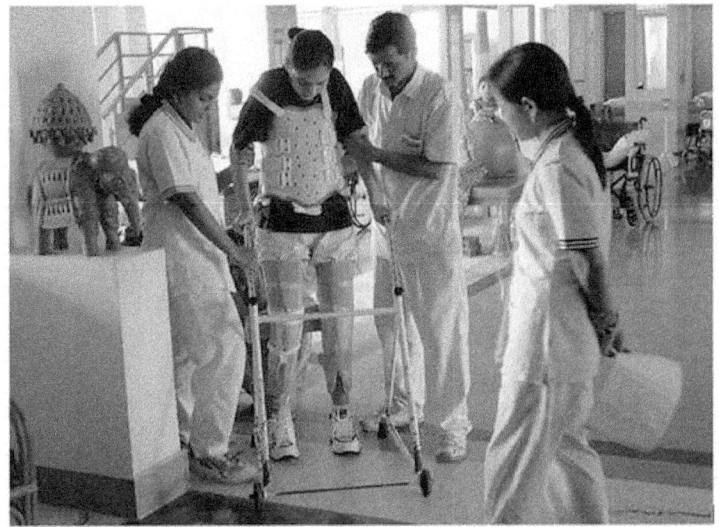

Gait training is a type of physical therapy. It can help improve your ability to stand and walk. Your doctor may recommend gait training if you've had an illness or injury that affects your ability to get around. It may help you gain independence in walking, even if you need an adaptive device.

Gait training can help:

- strengthen your muscles and joints
- improve your balance and posture
- build your endurance
- develop your muscle memory
- retrain your legs for repetitive motion
- lower your risk of falls, while increasing your mobility

It may also lower your risk of other illnesses, such as heart disease and osteoporosis, by increasing your physical activity and mobility. Choosing gait training over immobility may help protect and improve your overall health.

A doctor may recommend gait training if a patient has lost ability to walk due to an injury, illness, or other health condition. For example, the following conditions can lead to difficulties with walking:

- spinal cord injuries
- broken legs or pelvis
- joint injuries or replacements
- lower limb amputations
- strokes or neurological disorders
- muscular dystrophy or other musculoskeletal disorders

A patient is to start gait training as soon as possible after an injury or illness that affects their ability to walk. They may recommend other forms of physical therapy and treatments too. The patient must be healthy enough for physical activity and movement before they begin. Their joints must also be strong enough to support gait training.

The process is similar to other physical therapies. It often involves machines that help a patient walk safely. Therapists may also assist you in gait training exercises. They can help support a patient's bodyweight, provide stability, and offer other assistance.

Gait training commonly involves walking on a treadmill and completing muscle strengthening activities. A patient may wear a harness while walking on the treadmill or doing other exercises. The therapist may also ask the patient to practice stepping over objects, lifting their legs, sitting down, standing up, or other activities.

The type, intensity, and duration of training will depend on the patient's specific diagnosis and physical abilities.

ORTHOTICS

As we age, changes in the shape of our feet, the support of our ligaments in the feet, and previous injuries, can cause strain and pain. This is where a custom orthotic is a good idea to provide the needed support for your feet.

Orthotic inserts allow the feet and lower legs to function at their highest potential. Orthotics can decrease pain, alleviate pressure, and increase stability in an unstable joint. In addition, orthotics are used to treat specific pathologies such as diabetes, plantar fasciitis, hammer toes, heel spurs, and arthritis. Our techniques ensure that our orthotics fit the contours of your feet allowing for maximum support, comfort and function.

Although custom orthotics are more expensive than off-the-shelf devices, they last much longer and provide more support or correction.

If a patient suffers from the conditions below, then they can benefit from custom orthotics and physical therapy treatments.

- **Plantar fasciitis**, a common painful inflammation of the sole of the foot towards the heel, most easily recognized by its tendency to cause pain first thing in the morning
- **Arthritis**, which often affects different joints of the foot
- **Diabetes**, which interferes with circulation in the feet, requiring custom shoe modifications or custom-built footwear to alleviate pressure points
- **Metatarsalgia**, a painful foot disorder that affects the bones and joints at the ball of the foot
- **Heel spurs**, a growth of dense tissue or bone growing out of the calcaneous bone on the heel. This is due to excessive pressure on this region from changes in walking

Other potentially treatable conditions include patellofemoral knee pain, shin splints, achilles tendonitis, and bunions, as well as numerous systemic pathologies that (like diabetes) affect the function of the lower limbs.

PAIN MANAGEMENT

Physical Therapy for Pain Management

Physical therapy is used to alleviate sources of chronic pain, including:

- Osteoarthritis
- Fibromyalgia
- Chronic headaches
- Rheumatoid arthritis
- Neuropathic pain (pain caused by injury to tissues or nerves)

One of the goals of physical therapy, says Watson, is "to help chronic pain patients become stronger, because they're usually weak from not moving."

As a chronic pain treatment, physical therapy can teach people how to move safely and functionally in ways that they haven't been able to for quite a while, Watson adds.

Physical Therapy: Chronic Pain Treatment Options

Physical therapy involves a number of different types of pain management methods, says Watson, including:

- Massage
- Manipulation of joints and bones
- Manual therapy using hands or tools on soft tissue
- Cold laser therapy to alleviate inflammation and pain and release endorphins.
- Microcurrent stimulation, which emits alpha waves into the brain and increase serotonin and dopamine to alleviate pain naturally
- Movement therapy and exercise

Within each of these categories, there's much that a physical therapist has to offer as far as variety of treatments. Exercise may involve walking on a treadmill or swimming in a pool, depending on the person's pain and physical abilities.

A physical therapist works with each patient to understand his or her particular pain — what causes it and what can be done to manage it. This is the kind of attention that a regular doctor doesn't often have the time to give, but a physical therapist can ask questions and talk about pain issues as you are going through your exercise routine.

How Physical Therapy Helps Chronic Pain

Exercising for just 30 minutes a day on at least three or four days a week will help you with chronic pain management by increasing:

- Strength in the muscles
- Endurance
- Stability in the joints
- Flexibility in the muscles and joints

Keeping a consistent exercise routine will also help control chronic pain. Regular therapeutic exercise will help you maintain the ability to move and function physically, rather than becoming disabled by your chronic pain.

Physical therapy tackles the physical side of the inflammation, stiffness, and soreness with exercise, manipulation, and massage, but it also works to help the body heal itself by encouraging the production of the body's natural pain-relieving chemicals. This two-pronged approach is what helps make physical therapy so effective as a chronic pain treatment.

Pain Management: Finding the Right Combination

The less you move, the more pain you'll experience. Conversely, the more safe, therapeutic activity and exercise you get — and the more you learn how to exercise to accommodate your pain, the less pain you'll feel and the more you'll be able to function on a daily basis.

While physical therapy can be extremely effective against chronic pain, says Watson, it's important to understand that physical therapy is part of a combination approach to resolving chronic pain.

Watson recommends nutritional supplements, **heat and cold therapy,** and even transcutaneous electrical nerve stimulation (TENS) therapy as good additional pain management options along with physical therapy. He notes that it's important to work not just with a physical therapist, but also with a medical doctor who can prescribe any necessary medications. A clinical psychologist and a pharmacist are also important members of a pain management team, says Watson. Put all these components together to find the most effective chronic pain treatment for you.

RANGE OF MOTION

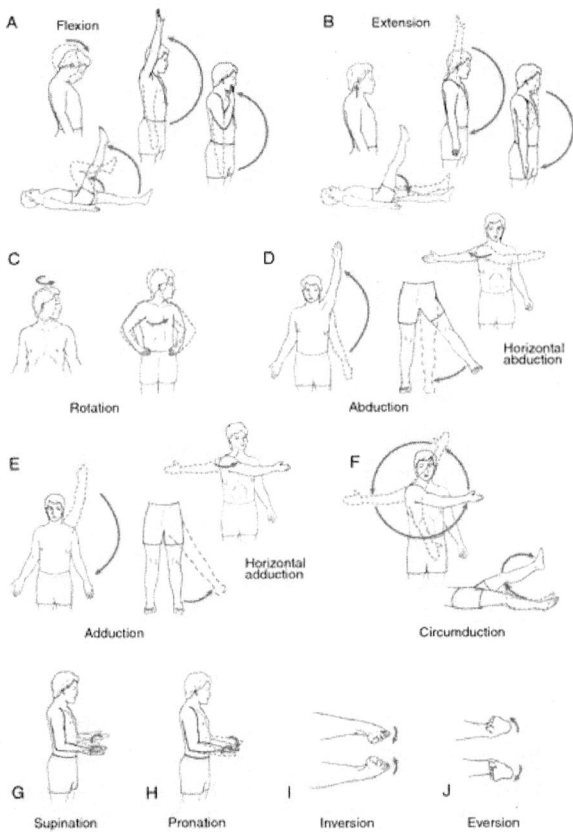

Definition of Range of Motion

Range of Motion is the measurement of movement around a specific joint or body part.

Let's say a soccer player named Jane has torn a ligament in her knee and is working with a physical therapist to try and regain her range of motion. Initially, she was rather limited in her movement, but since performing the stretching exercises regularly, the therapist has confirmed that her range of motion has been getting closer to her pre-injury level of functioning.

Importance Of Flexibility

In order for a joint to have full range of motion, it must have good flexibility. Each joint has its own level of flexibility, expressed in degrees. **Flexibility** is the range of motion around a joint, and can refer to ligaments, tendons, muscles, bones, and joints. If a joint has good range of motion then it would be able to move in all planes and directions permitted to that joint. For example, the elbow, which is a hinged joint, only permits movement in one direction, but it should provide full range of motion from extension to flexion.

Although flexibility is the most neglected fitness component, it is important for general health, injury prevention, and even sports performance. Factors that may contribute to a lack in the range of motion could be pain, swelling, and stiffness in the joints, side effects common in arthritis, rheumatoid arthritis, and osteoarthritis. Injuries can have lasting effects on how freely a joint moves. Other factors that can determine one's flexibility are joint structure, muscles, tendons, ligaments, fat tissue, body temperature, activity level, gender, age, and genetics.

Types of Range of Motion

There are three primary types of exercises specific to range of motion. **Passive range of motion** is typically practiced on a joint that is inactive. The physical therapist may use this exercise on a client who is paralyzed or unable to mobilize a specific joint. This type of exercise can help prevent stiffness from occurring. During this exercise the patient does not perform any movement, while the therapist stretches the patient's soft tissues.

Active-assistive range of motion exercises are more progressive, intended for the client to perform movement around the joint, with some manual assistance from the physical therapist or from a strap or band. These exercises can often feel painful, and the muscles can feel weak. Increasing range of motion with these exercises should be a gradual advancement.

Active range of motion exercises are highly independent, performed solely by the client. The physical therapist's role may be simply to provide verbal cues.

Active vs Passive

Your active and passive range of motion may be very different, not only from each other, but also at the joints themselves. Active range of motion means you move a joint through its range of motion, or ROM. Passive range of motion involves someone else moving a joint for you. Anytime you are moving your body, you are using active ROM. An example of passive ROM is if a doctor is testing a joint, such as the shoulder, and is moving it for you without your assistance.

Importance of Each

Active ROM is what you work with everyday and tends to be the type of ROM that concerns most people. If you have limited active ROM, you may have trouble lifting your arms overhead for exercising or putting away groceries, for example. It could also limit performance during sporting activities and thus increase the chance of injury. Passive ROM is not a concern for everyone, however. It is significant if you have a long-term or permanent change to your body, such as being in a wheelchair. You may not be able to move your joints, but having a nurse or therapist do it for you helps maintain ROM and can reduce pain or dysfunction. It is also used a lot for physical therapy if you have an injury.

How to Improve ROM

Active and passive ROM can be improved through stretching and even strengthening exercises. Dynamic stretches, such as arm circles, or pulling one knee at a time to your chest in a standing position, take strength and flexibility. It is good for warming up before a sport performance or exercise. Static stretches where you hold a stretch can improve both active and passive ROM. These are the stretches you do after a workout when your muscles are warmed up. Holding a stretch 15 seconds or longer can show greater improvements to your active ROM than shorter stretches, according to researchers from School of Health Sciences, University of Sunderland, United Kingdom, who published a study in the "British Journal of Sports Medicine."

Factors Affecting ROM

There are many factors that can affect both active and passive ROM. Your lifestyle is a major contributing factor. If you are sedentary, or perform repetitive tasks throughout the day, you may have limited ROM. Injury or a chronic condition, such as arthritis, could also affect both active and passive ROM. Your body size can also limit ROM. If you are overweight, excess skin and fat could impede your movement. As you lose weight, however, you will notice that both active and passive ROM improves.

SPINAL CORD

Spinal Cord Overview

C1 Cervical spinal nerve roots C1 - C7 correspond with upper aspects of vertebral bodies.

Bone notch at the base of the neck is C7.

C8 Sensation of C7 nerve is for the middle finger.

T1

C8 and lower spinal nerve roots leave below the corresponding vertebral body.

T4 Sensation of T4 spinal nerve is approximately level with the nipple line.

T6 Sensation of T6 spinal nerve root is approximately level with the bottom of the sternum.

T10 Sensation of T10 spinal nerve root is approximately level with the abdomen.

T12 Sensation of T12 spinal nerve root is approximately level with the pubic bone.

L1

The spinal cord ends approximately between L1 & L2.

The sensations of lumbar nerves are over the legs.

Sacral cord segments (S1-S5 "cauda equina") are level with T12-L1 vertebrae.

L5

S1

The sacral vertebrae are fused to make up the sacrum.

S3 Sensation of S3,S4 & S5 nerves is the perineal (genital) area.

S5

The coccygeal vertebrae are fused to make the coccyx or "tail bone".

Coc1 Sensation to coccygeal area.

Spinal Cord Nerve Roots

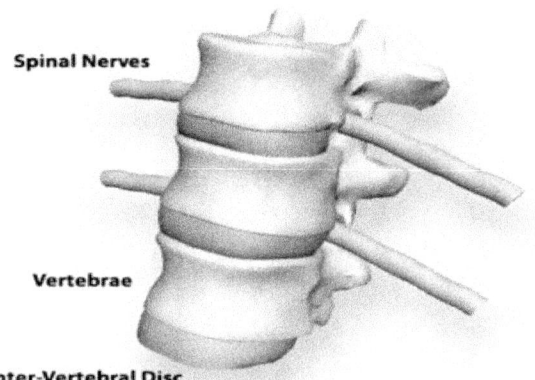

Spinal Nerves

Vertebrae

Inter-Vertebral Disc

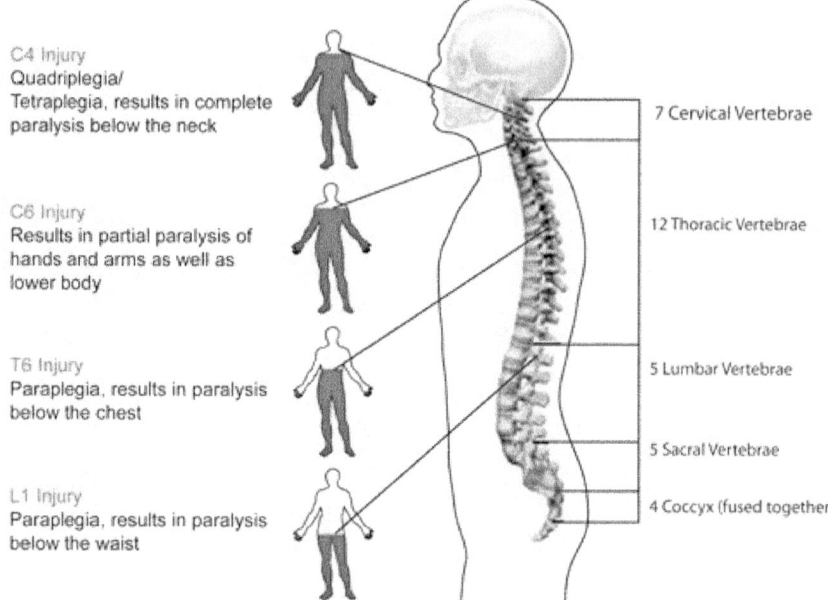

C4 Injury
Quadriplegia/
Tetraplegia, results in complete
paralysis below the neck

C6 Injury
Results in partial paralysis of
hands and arms as well as
lower body

T6 Injury
Paraplegia, results in paralysis
below the chest

L1 Injury
Paraplegia, results in paralysis
below the waist

7 Cervical Vertebrae

12 Thoracic Vertebrae

5 Lumbar Vertebrae

5 Sacral Vertebrae

4 Coccyx (fused together)

The spinal cord is connected to the brain and is about the diameter of a human finger. From the brain the spinal cord descends down the middle of the back and is surrounded and protected by the bony vertebral column. The spinal cord is surrounded by a clear fluid called cerebral spinal fluid (CSF), that acts as a cushion to protect the delicate nerve tissues against damage from banging against the inside of the vertebrae.

The anatomy of the spinal cord itself, consists of millions of nerve fibres which transmit electrical information to and from the limbs, trunk and organs of the body, back to and from the brain. The nerves which exit the spinal cord in the upper section, the neck, control breathing and the arms. The nerves which exit the spinal cord in the mid and lower section of the back, control the trunk and legs, as well as bladder, bowel and sexual function.

The nerves which carry information from the brain to muscles are called motor neurons. The nerves which carry information from the body back to the brain are called sensory neurons.

Sensory neurons carry information to the brain about skin temperature, touch, pain and joint position.

The brain and spinal cord are referred to as the central nervous system (CNS), whilst the nerves connecting the spinal cord to the body are referred to as the peripheral nervous system (PNS).

Ascending and Descending Spinal Tracts

The nerves within the spinal cord are grouped together in different bundles called ascending and descending tracts.

- Ascending tracts within the spinal cord carry sensory information from the body upwards to the brain such as touch, skin temperature, pain and joint position.
- Descending tracts within the spinal cord carry information from the brain downwards to initiate movement and control body functions.

Spinal Nerves

Nerves called the spinal nerves or nerve root, branch off the spinal cord and pass out through a hole in each of the vertebrae called the foramen. These nerves carry information from the spinal cord to the rest of the body, and from the body back up to the brain.

There are four main groups of spinal nerves, which exit different levels of the spinal cord.

These are in descending order down the vertebral column:

- **Cervical Nerves "C":** (nerves in the neck) supply movement and feeling to the arms, neck and upper trunk. Also control breathing.
- **Thoracic Nerves "T":** (nerves in the upper back) supply the trunk and abdomen.
- **Lumbar Nerves "L" and Sacral Nerves "S":** (nerves in the lower back) supply the legs, the bladder, bowel and sexual organs.

Spinal Cord Level Numbering System

The spinal nerves carry information to and from different levels (segments) in the spinal cord. Both the nerves and the segments in the spinal cord are numbered in a similar way to the vertebrae. The point at which the spinal cord ends is called the conus medullaris, and is the terminal end of the spinal cord. It occurs near lumbar nerves L1 and L2. After the spinal cord terminates, the spinal nerves continue as a bundle of nerves called the cauda equina. The upper end of the conus medullaris is usually not well defined.

There are 31 pairs of spinal nerves which branch off from the spinal cord. In the cervical region of the spinal cord, the spinal nerves exit above the vertebrae. A change occurs with the C7 vertebra however where the C8 spinal nerve exits the vertebra below the C7 vertebra. Therefore, there is an 8th cervical spinal nerve even though there is no 8th cervical vertebra. From the 1st thoracic vertebra downwards, all spinal nerves exit below their equivalent numbered vertebrae.

The spinal nerves which leave the spinal cord are numbered according to the vertebra at which they exit the spinal column. So, the spinal nerve T4, exits the spinal column through the foramen in the 4th thoracic vertebra. The spinal nerve L5 leaves the spinal cord from the conus medullaris, and travels along the cauda equina until it exits the 5th lumbar vertebra.

The level of the spinal cord segments do not relate exactly to the level of the vertebral bodies i.e. damage to the bone at a particular level e.g. L5 vertebrae does not necessarily mean damage to the spinal cord at the same spinal nerve level.

ULTRASOUND

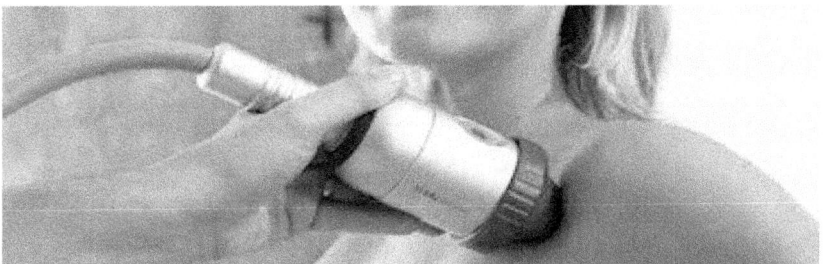

Ultrasound is a therapeutic modality that has been used by physical therapists since the 1940s. Ultrasound is applied using a round-headed wand or probe that is put in direct contact with the patient's skin. Ultrasound gel is used on all surfaces of the head in order to reduce friction and assist in the transmission of the ultrasonic waves. Therapeutic ultrasound is in the frequency range of about 0.8-3.0 MHz.

The waves are generated by a piezoelectric effect caused by the vibration of crystals within the head of the wand/probe. The sound waves that pass through the skin cause a vibration of the local tissues. This vibration or cavitation can cause a deep heating locally though usually no sensation of heat will be felt by the patient. In situations where a heating effect is not desirable, such as a fresh injury with acute inflammation, the ultrasound can be pulsed rather than continuously transmitted.

Ultrasound can produce many effects other than just the potential heating effect. It has been shown to cause increases in tissue relaxation, local blood flow, and scar tissue breakdown. The effect of the increase in local blood flow can be used to help reduce local swelling and chronic inflammation, and, according to some studies, promote bone fracture healing. The intensity or power density of the ultrasound can be adjusted depending on the desired effect. A greater power density (measured in watt/cm^2 is often used in cases where scar tissue breakdown is the goal.

Ultrasound can also be used to achieve phonophoresis. This is a non-invasive way of administering medications to tissues below the skin; perfect for patients who are uncomfortable with injections. With this technique, the ultrasonic energy forces the medication through the skin.

Cortisone, used to reduce inflammation, is one of the more commonly used substances delivered in this way.

A typical ultrasound treatment will take from 3-5 minutes depending on the size of the area being treated. In cases where scar tissue breakdown is the goal, this treatment time can be much longer. During the treatment the head of the ultrasound probe is kept in constant motion. If kept in constant motion, the patient should feel no discomfort at all. If the probe is held in one place for more than just a few seconds, a buildup of the sound energy can result which can become uncomfortable. Interestingly, if there is even a very minor break in a bone in the area that is close to the surface, a sharp pain may be felt. This occurs as the sound waves get trapped between the two parts of the break and build up until becoming painful. In this way ultrasound can often be used as a fairly accurate tool for diagnosing minor fractures that may not be obvious on x-ray.

Some conditions treated with ultrasound include tendonitis (or tendinitis if you prefer), non-acute joint swelling, muscle spasm, and even Peyronie's Disease (to break down the scar tissue). Contraindications of ultrasound include local malignancy, metal implants below the area being treated, local acute infection, vascular abnormalities, and directly on the abdomen of pregnant women. It is also contraindicated to apply ultrasound directly over active epiphyseal regions (growth plates) in children, over the spinal cord in the area of a laminectomy, or over the eyes, skull, or testes.

www.ingramcontent.com/pod-product-compliance
Lightning Source LLC
Chambersburg PA
CBHW070133210526
45170CB00013B/904